One in six people over the age of 80 develop
dementia – including both our fathers.
This book is dedicated to them – and to our
mothers, who have shared their journey.

Can I tell you about...?

The "Can I tell you about...?" series offers simple introductions to a range of limiting conditions. Friendly characters invite readers to learn about their experiences of living with a particular condition and how they would like to be helped and supported. These books serve as excellent starting points for family and classroom discussions.

other books in the "Can I tell you about...?" series

Can I tell you about Asperger Syndrome?
A guide for friends and family
Jude Welton
Foreword by Elizabeth Newson
Illustrated by Jane Telford
ISBN 978 1 84310 206 9
eISBN 978 1 84642 422 9

Can I tell you about Epilepsy?
A guide for friends, family and professionals
Kate Lambert
Illustrated by Scott Hellier
ISBN 978 1 84905 309 9
eISBN 978 0 85700 648 6

Can I tell you about Selective Mutism?
A guide for friends, family and professionals
Maggie Johnson and Alison Wintgens
Illustrated by Robyn Gallow
ISBN 978 1 84905 289 4
eISBN 978 0 85700 611 0

of related interest

Dementia – Support for Family and Friends
Dave Pulsford and Rachel Thompson
ISBN 978 1 84905 243 6
eISBN 978 0 85700 504 5
Part of the Support for Family and Friends series

Telling Tales About Dementia
Experiences of Caring
Edited by Lucy Whitman
Foreword by Joanna Trollope
ISBN 978 1 84310 941 9
eISBN 978 0 85700 017 0

Contents

Introduction

In the early stage of dementia, some people may be able to give insights into their experience. But once the condition has advanced, it would not be possible for someone with dementia to tell their story in the way Jack does. Jack wouldn't really be able to reflect on his condition or analyse it or find the words to describe what he was thinking or feeling. So with this little book, I would ask you to "suspend disbelief", and listen to the words that someone with dementia might tell you if they could.

Living with dementia is a challenge for those with the condition, and for those who care for them. I hope that Jack's words will help to show how behaviours that might seem puzzling and bizarre make sense if we appreciate what it really means to lose your memory, and lose your ability to think clearly, to reason and to communicate. If we step into Jack's shoes, we can try to understand what life might be like for someone with dementia. If we understand what it might be like, we are much more able to help.

What can be done to help? Medication can temporarily slow the progress of certain forms of dementia. Being physically active and keeping the brain engaged by doing things such as crossword puzzles may have a positive effect. There are many ways we can structure the environment to make life easier. But it is the way we relate to and behave towards the person with dementia which has by far the biggest impact on their quality of life.

We need to respect the person as an individual, ensuring that they continue to feel cared for and valued. This will mean acknowledging a reality that may not (initially at least) make sense to us. People with dementia lose the ability to remember new information, so they may make sense of what is happening now by using the only memories they still have – those of the distant past. You may think it is silly for an elderly person to worry about his children getting to school on time, and may think it is doing him a favour to point this out to him. But in this sort of situation, pointing out that he is "mistaken" can be counterproductive: it serves to increase distress, not reduce it.

Once we accept that what is true for them is true for them, we can avoid fruitless arguments of the "Oh yes it is/Oh no it isn't" variety, and life can become happier for the person with dementia and for their carer.

Even if we know (in our fully functioning brains) that what the person with dementia is thinking is not "accurate", it helps to go with their flow, and play along as if we "know what they mean". This can be a difficult thing to accept or do, but it makes all the difference to their well-being (and ours). I remember watching my husband appearing to have an animated conversation with his mother, who was in the late stages of dementia with Lewy bodies (see p. 44). If you listened to the words they spoke they made no sense, but there was a real sense of a conversation going on with nods, and nudges, and hand pats and conspiratorial smiles. My husband had entered into his Mum's world, and they had connected: she seemed to be enjoying a really good chat.

Learning how to listen and observe, finding ways to reassure or distract, learning not to contradict or confront but to steer the conversation to topics that make the person relaxed and happy, understanding and coping with unusual behaviour caused by problems with reasoning or memory, finding satisfying activities they can enjoy, keeping them safe and "on track" (reminding them gently what day it is if that are confused, for example)... it all needs tolerance, creativity, stamina, a sense of humour and heaps of patience! It can be emotionally and physically exhausting. But it's not all doom and gloom: it is still possible to have fun and laughter.

If you are caring for someone with dementia, make sure you also take care of yourself, by seeking help, support and guidance, by sharing the caring, and by taking breaks. Caring for someone with dementia is not something you can do alone. Check out the organisations on pp. 46–48, and don't be afraid to ask for help.

Everyone's story will be unique. The way someone experiences dementia will depend on various factors, including the type of dementia they have, the type of personality they have, and the quality of support they receive. But I hope that Jack's story will help you understand what the experience of dementia is like for someone you care for, so that you can make a positive impact on their life.

Now, over to Jack...

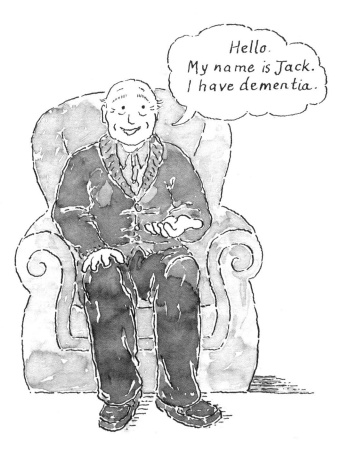

"Losing my memory is at the heart of it all. I can't remember anything new, and old memories are disappearing too."

"I've had dementia for quite a few years. I've got Alzheimer's disease, the most common form of dementia. There are other types of dementia,[1] but they all damage the brain so that it can't work the way it used to.

It's strange: I can sometimes still remember things that happened long, long ago – but I can't remember what someone said or did two minutes ago. Nothing sticks. And distant memories have begun to disappear too. Now I can't understand things I used to understand easily. I find it hard to make decisions and to carry out everyday tasks. I have problems with communicating too.

It's not surprising that it affects my mood. The world doesn't make sense any more. I sometimes feel frightened, confused, angry and frustrated if I can't remember what I was going to say, or I can't understand what's happening or remember who people are.

I'll tell you about the way dementia has affected me over the last few years. Some of the problems, like wandering, stopped after a while. Others, such as memory loss, have got worse.

I'll tell you about things that have helped me feel good and have helped me connect with the 'me' I used to be. Things like reminiscing about football, watching old films and singing songs from the old days.

I've had a good, long life. I served in World War 2. I used to run my own business. I took pride in looking after my wife and family. Now I have to rely on other people to look after me. But I'm still an individual, who needs respect. I'm still Jack."

---

1 Other types of dementia are described on pp. 43–45.

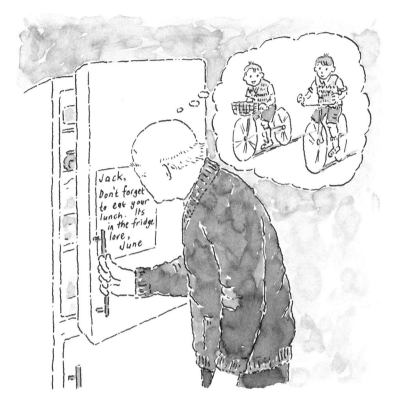

"I used to cycle to the shop to collect groceries for Mum and Dad. Past things like this don't always feel like 'a memory'. They feel like now."

"The first sign that something was wrong was when I had lapses in my memory. At first my wife and I thought it was just a bit of forgetfulness – you expect that when you're 80 years old! But then I started to get confused. I often couldn't remember what day it was, I kept losing things, got lost myself, and I couldn't remember what people said to me. It was scary. We went to see my doctor. It turned out I had Alzheimer's disease.

The way memory loss happens is slightly different depending on the type of dementia you have, but with Alzheimer's it seems to start with the brain no longer being able to take in and remember new information. I'd forget things that had just happened, even though I could clearly remember things I did as a boy.

As time has passed, I have forgotten more and more. Gradually I am forgetting everything I have learned since childhood. Because of the changes going on in my brain, I will unlearn everything I've learned, mainly in reverse order.[2]

You can think of it as happening a bit like this: imagine writing today's date on a blackboard, and then writing every year counting backwards to the year I was born – 2012, 2011, 2010, 2009... all the way back to 1923. Now imagine someone taking a blackboard rubber and wiping out everything starting with 2012 and going back to 1923... The last memories to remain are the earliest ones."

---

2   This "most recent to most distant" progression in memory loss explains why some people in the late stage of dementia start using the language they learned when they were a child, even if they moved abroad later and learned a new language.

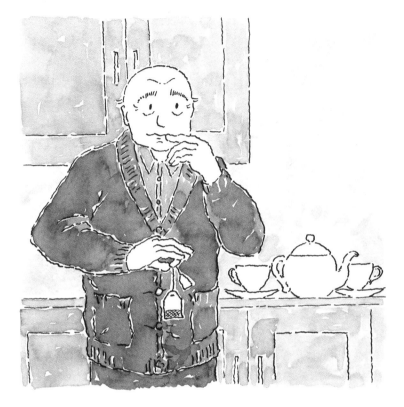

"Even making a cup of tea got beyond me."

"Until you start losing your memory, you take it for granted. But to live your life, and make sense of things, you need your memory. Memory isn't just about remembering facts and figures. It's what lets you remember people's names and faces, remember where you live, remember how to get home – even remember when to eat or how to get dressed. You even need your memory to remember who you are.

Your memory is like the store of everything you've ever done or learned throughout your life. And because of my Alzheimer's disease, that store is gradually being emptied.

I live life moment by moment, without memory to bind all the moments together and give them meaning. I've lost sense of where I am in time, so I'm losing the future as well as the past. Losing my memory stopped me from being able to plan things, or look forward to things, or keep track of things I'm doing.

If you can't remember new things, you can't remember what's just happened or what's meant to happen next. When we got a new TV, I could never learn how to switch it on – however many times my son showed me. I'd forget step 1 by the time he was on step 2.

It's not just that I can't learn new things. I've forgotten how to do things I always used to do. I used to love cooking, but eventually cooking was no longer possible. I might put the pan on, and then forget about it. I switched on the gas and forgot to light it. It was dangerous."

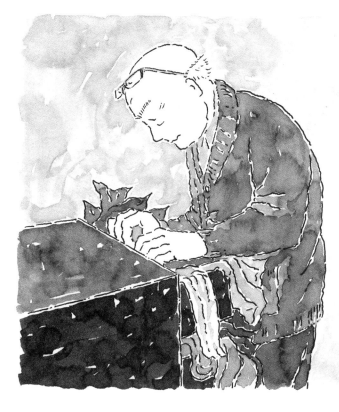

"I kept forgetting where I put things, so I put them in a 'safe' place. Then I couldn't remember where I'd put them."

"It's normal to become a bit more forgetful as you get older. But with dementia the forgetfulness gets worse and makes life really difficult. I used to have a great memory. I had to: I ran my own business, and was responsible for lots of people. But I kept forgetting where I'd put things. At first I blamed my wife. I thought she was hiding things. I suppose I couldn't face the fact that it was me.

I knew something was really wrong one day when I was in town shopping with my wife. We'd separated and were meant to meet up at the car, but I couldn't remember where we'd parked – even though we've parked in the same place for years. I've never managed to learn how to use one of those mobile phones, so I couldn't phone her. I was completely lost. A stranger helped me.

In my work I had to analyse new information and make decisions very quickly, but I started to find that really difficult. That made me very anxious, and I started to lose interest in things.

Losing my memory means I can't make decisions, make judgements or think about consequences. To make decisions and make judgements, you have to be able to hold lots of information in your head at once and analyse it. My brain can't do that any more. For example, I can no longer judge whether my behaviour is appropriate or not. I might behave in a way you think is rude. I always prided myself on having good manners. I would never mean to be rude. Please understand that."

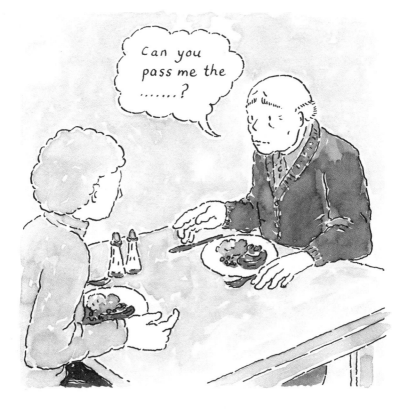

"Quite early on, I'd often forget what things were called! That was really frustrating."

"My ability to use words to communicate gradually got worse. At first, I'd forget the names of things. Like 'toothbrush'. I knew what it was, and I knew what to do with it, but just couldn't remember the name for it. At that stage I could understand most of what people said to me, but I often couldn't find the word I was looking for when I wanted to say something. It was very frustrating.

Conversations became difficult, because I couldn't remember what someone had just said. Or what question they had asked. Or what I'd just said. Sometimes I didn't recognise who was talking to me, even though they seemed to know who I was. Even if I was watching a football match on the TV, I couldn't talk about it much, because I couldn't remember what had just happened or what the score was.

Later, I started to talk less. I didn't know how to start a conversation, and just said little snippets of sentences. By this stage, I often couldn't understand what people were talking about.

In the late stages, I may stop talking. I might not be able to tell you if I'm in pain, or uncomfortable, or what I'm upset about – or even that I can't see properly with my glasses. So you may need to work those things out without the help of my words.

Some people in the home I live in now don't say words. Some just make sounds. Especially if they are distressed or confused – they make upset noises. And they might hit out. Imagine if you wanted to tell someone to 'Get off me!', but didn't have the words. How would you communicate that?"

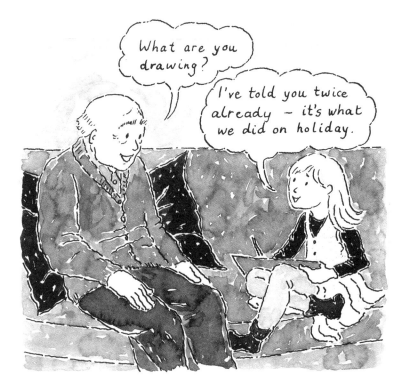

"If I ask the same question over and over again, it's because nothing new sticks in my brain."

"One of the first things people noticed was that I started to repeat myself. That can be pretty annoying for other people, but it wasn't great for me either! If you can't remember what's been said, and you sense someone is exasperated with you, it makes you feel stupid and sometimes angry.

When I began to feel frightened and adrift in the world, I asked my wife the same things over and over again, for reassurance. I couldn't remember asking the question, and couldn't remember the answer. It must have driven her up the wall, but she tried to find an answer that satisfied me. She sometimes wrote the answer on a card and pointed it out to me.

Occasionally, I use bad language. I never used to swear, but I've had outbursts when I've said really bad words. Alzheimer's disease has been stripping away my ability to think about what I'm saying or to consider the effect of what I say. I don't know how to be tactful any more. Please remember, if I say something rude, it's not because I mean to. It's all part of my condition.

I sometimes talk as if a past event is happening now – which it is in my mind! Sometimes people think I'm talking rubbish if I say, 'I'm late for work,' or 'Turn those lights out! There's a bombing raid on the way!' That might seem nonsense, but it's not nonsense to me. Sometimes a memory seems to surface in my brain from long ago, and it feels as if it's happening now. If people contradict what I'm saying, I don't like it. It makes me confused and distressed. "

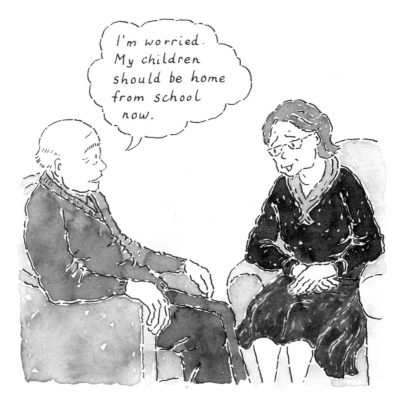

"Past and present have become the same to me. My feelings might link with a past experience that feels as if it's happening now."

"It's understandable that dementia has affected my mood. I used to be pretty easy-going, but since I've had Alzheimer's disease, I've been angry, sad, withdrawn, apathetic, confused, anxious and suspicious. Sometimes my feelings are all mixed up, and sometimes they swing from one to another. I might be upset one moment, and then forget what I was upset about. I sometimes feel worries that are to do with things that happened long ago – but it feels as if they're happening now.

I felt anxious in the early stages when I was aware that other people remembered things that I couldn't. Can you imagine what it feels like when other people seem to know what you've been doing, but you don't? Imagine what it's like when someone asks you where you've put the house keys, and insists that they saw you with the house keys, and you can't remember seeing them. You feel muddled up and worthless.

My emotions aren't always negative. I used to enjoy it when someone went for a good walk with me. When my wife sits stroking my hand and talking gently, I feel comforted and content. When we have a sing-song together, I feel energised and happy. When I watch the fish swimming in the fish tank, I feel calm. When I'm eating a lovely meal of chicken and chips, or my wife gives me my favourite sweets, I feel pleasure.

I don't have feelings of guilt or shame. Before I had dementia I would have been ashamed of some of the things I do now, like swearing. But to feel shame or guilt, you have to be able to analyse and reflect on your behaviour, and my brain can't do that any more."

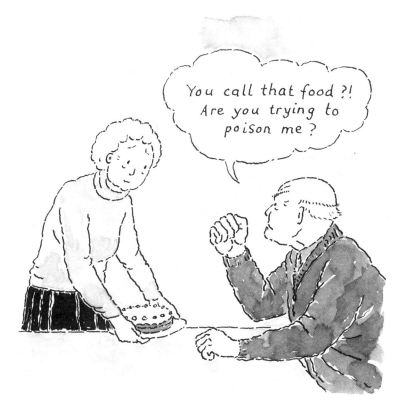

"I've been suspicious and aggressive towards my wife. I never was before. It's horrible. It's caused by my problems understanding what's going on."

"Even when I've lost the ability to say what I'm thinking and feeling, my feelings show in my body language and expression, and in the things I do. If I can't tell you what a problem is, you'll need to try to work out the meaning behind my behaviour. That can help you to deal with any challenges.

I used to pace about if I felt anxious or agitated. I used to follow my wife about, and walk to the door and back, over and over again. It helped if someone offered to take me for a walk. I usually felt better for the exercise and I often forgot what I was upset about.

Sometimes I hide things away, even food. I get suspicious. Imagine what it would be like if you didn't know who was who – you might get very suspicious too. Sometimes I don't even recognise my wife.

I have been physically aggressive, which I *never* was before. If someone tries to stop me going where I want to go, or tries to make me move when I don't want to, I might get frightened and push them away or hit out. If someone talks to me in an angry voice, or I look at them and they remind me of someone who hurt me in the past, I might feel threatened and lash out to protect myself.

Please understand that suspicion, fear and aggression are caused by the way my brain is misinterpreting what is happening, because of my problems with memory and understanding. Not everyone with dementia gets aggressive. But if they do, carers need to try to understand and predict triggers for aggression, and take steps to keep everyone safe."

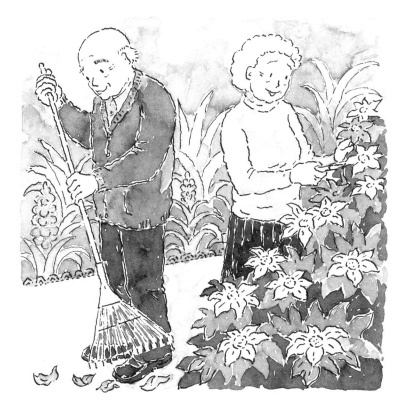

"It's good to keep doing things for as long as you can. Gardening with my wife, I enjoyed the exercise, the fresh air, the companionship, and the sense of achievement."

"I'm gradually forgetting how to do things such as getting dressed and undressed, washing, shaving, cooking – even going to the toilet and eating. Mainly these skills are getting lost in reverse order, so that in the end I may not know or do any more than I did as a baby.

Early on, my wife encouraged me to make lists and keep a diary of things to do. She put reminder notes on the fridge. She put picture labels on the drawers to remind me where the cutlery was and so on. This all helped me keep on track.

We did household chores together, so my wife could show me what to. I would wash up, while my wife dried the dishes. She encouraged me to do things like making the bed, folding the washing and working in the garden. It's good to keep doing things for as long as you can, because it's good to feel capable and useful.

I started to have 'accidents' going to the toilet. Sometimes I got confused, and mistook the wastepaper basket for the toilet, especially at night. That was very difficult for my wife to cope with. Then she took away the basket, and left the light on in the loo, so that I was drawn towards the light if I woke up. That helped.

In the morning, my wife used to lay out my clothes in the order I put them on. That helped me to dress independently. Later on she had to pass me my clothes in the right order. Now the carers help me to dress.

Even though I'm losing these skills, and need lots of help, I like being gently encouraged to try to do things as long as I'm able to. I can still brush my hair if someone starts me off!"

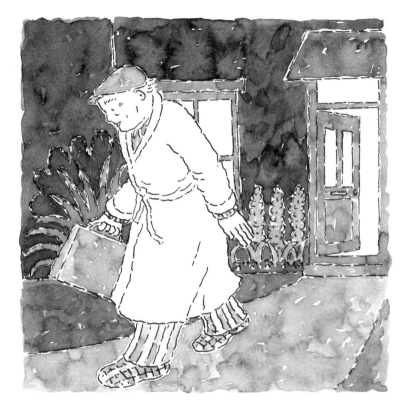

"I went through a stage of getting up and dressed in the night. It was a real challenge for my family while it lasted."

"I've always been an active person. And as my dementia took hold, I often became restless. I had the urge to pace about.

Sometimes I'd go to front door, and my wife would ask where I was going. I'd say: 'Work, of course. That business can't run without me.' She learned that it didn't help to tell me I stopped work ages ago. Instead she'd say, 'It's OK. James (our son) is on duty today. I really need you to help me work in the garden.' That usually satisfied me, and we'd go out and do some gardening.

I've had some trouble sleeping. If I wake in the night, I might think it's day time. I used to get dressed in the night sometimes. It was exhausting for my wife. She started putting away my day clothes at night, so I'd be less likely to think about getting dressed.

I went through a phase of getting very restless and confused in the evenings (it's called 'sundowning') and even went 'wandering' at night. One night the police found me: I'd found my way back to my old office! I didn't realise anything was wrong, so it didn't worry me, but it was a nightmare for my family.

I'm not aware when I'm putting myself at risk, so other people have to make sure I'm safe. My son fitted alarms so my wife knew when I got out of bed. They changed the house locks. They put a 'dementia alert' card with emergency contact numbers, and even a tracking device, in my jacket."

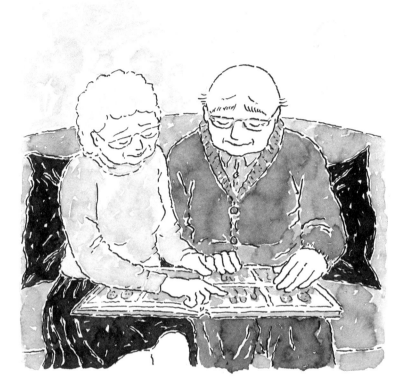

"My wife made a memory scrapbook. It helped
bring back old times, so we could have a bit
of a talk and a laugh about the old days."

"As my dementia progresses, I have become less and less able to start a conversation, so please help by starting conversations for me. Looking at old photographs and objects from the past can help trigger memories of old times.

Please don't ask me complicated questions or ask me to make complex choices. Keep things simple when you speak to me. Speak clearly. Get my attention before you speak, and give me extra time to process your words.

Please don't whisper to other people in front of me. It might make me feel suspicious and threatened. I might think you are saying nasty things about me. And use a calm tone of voice. I feel frightened if you raise your voice. Please don't come up behind me and speak. That can feel shocking and frightening too.

Unless it's important for safety, please don't contradict me or correct me if I say something you might think is silly, just because you think it's not true. If I say, 'I've got to catch the train to London,' I might be thinking that 'now' is 50 years ago, and that I am on my way to a business meeting. So it is true – for me. It helps me feel better about myself if you appear to agree with me – even if you don't.

If I am sitting down, please sit or bend down to my level to talk whenever possible. It can feel intimidating to have someone standing over me. Don't talk over me as if I am not there – it's important to me to feel respected and included."

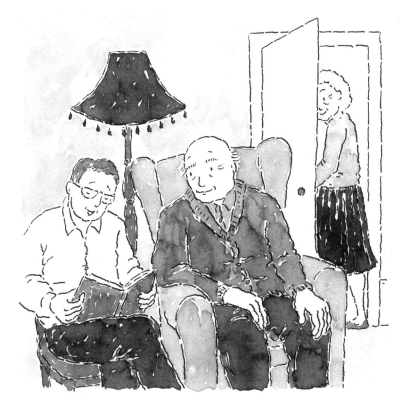

"My wife needed to take breaks, and it was good for me too. Sometimes my son used to read me my favourite poems."

"Caring for someone with dementia is tough, emotionally and physically. It's not possible to do it all by yourself. Don't be afraid to ask family, friends and neighbours to help out. There are lots of organisations and services to support you (see pp. 46–48).

As well as getting outside help, make sure you take regular breaks – or you'll damage your own health and won't be able to manage. You couldn't get a more loving person than my wife. We'd hardly spent a night apart in 60 years! But once my dementia started to take hold, she needed breaks. She had her 'special' time to herself each day. Sometimes she popped out to see friends, while someone stayed with me at home, or took me out. Occasionally she had a weekend away, while my son or daughter stayed with me. She came back home with her batteries recharged.

One of the most difficult points was when the time came for me to go into a care home. My wife said she'd never let it happen. But she shouldn't feel guilty. It had to happen. By that stage she was exhausted with my night wandering, and she had to keep an eye on me 24 hours a day, and had to do almost everything for me. She wasn't strong enough to keep going, and it was getting unsafe for both of us.

I'm well looked after here, and my family and friends visit me. When my wife visits, her smiling face lights up the room! She smiles more now that she's not exhausted by being responsible for me all the time, and we can spend quality time together."

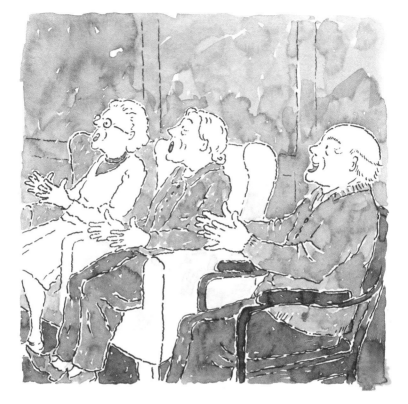

"Singing together is great fun. Even those of us who can't use words to have a conversation can remember the words and tunes of songs!"

"Activities are important. They stop me being bored. When I get bored, I get grumpy and agitated. But when it comes to activities, it's not one size fits all. I'm not just someone with dementia, I'm Jack, and I've got my own interests, likes and dislikes.

I've always loved gardening. I used to garden with my wife, and in the early stage of my dementia, my nephew sometimes took me to his allotment. I'd lost confidence, and was a bit worried about going, but I enjoyed it when I did. In the care home where I live now, I help look after the tomato plants in the greenhouse. I still love the smell of tomatoes, and it's good to feel I'm doing something useful.

Some people enjoy playing bingo. But I've never liked it. What I really enjoy is when we have a sing-song. We do movements as we sing, so we're exercising too. It's strange how I can remember the words from songs! Singing can sometimes trigger using spoken words too. It's a real highlight for me, and for lots of us.

Another highlight is what they call 'reminiscing' – thinking about the old times. That puts me in touch with the old 'me'. My daughter made me a memory box with photos and things. Rummaging through it can bring up memories, and make me smile. At our care home we've got what they call a 1950s room, with furniture and objects from the fifties, including an old radio, a typewriter and old toys like the ones we gave the kids. Sometimes we watch old war films or films of old football matches. We listen to the old band music too. I enjoy that. It takes me back."

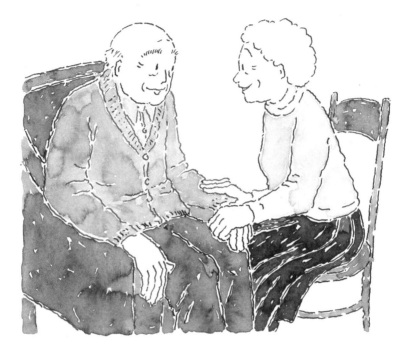

"Seeing a smiling face makes me feel good. My wife has a lovely smile. When she smiles, I smile too."

"As I lose the ability to understand the meaning of the words you say, the way you say them becomes especially important. The way you speak to me can make me feel scared or distressed, or it can make me feel safe and valued.

Your body language, your tone of voice and the expression on your face all have a powerful impact on the way I feel. Gentle touch, while you are speaking to me, is usually reassuring, and can help me feel connected to you. Sometimes if you sing to me gently it helps me relax. But be aware that I might not always feel that way.

When I don't understand what words mean, the only way I can judge whether I am safe and whether you are friendly or not is the *way* you talk and the *way* you behave towards me, and the *way* your expression looks. Smile please! It helps me to feel safe, secure and valued. It makes me feel a *person*.

Once facts have gone from my memory, it's feelings that remain. And even if I can't make sense of what you are saying, if you speak in a gentle, reassuring, happy way to me, it can make me feel good. It might be difficult for you to smile, especially if I am unresponsive, but it is important for me. I may still be able to 'pick up' on enthusiasm and caring humour.

Eventually, everything I've learned since babyhood may have disappeared from my memory – but even babies respond to a smile. Smile please. But remember that even though I may end up not knowing much more than I did as a child, I'm not a child, and I need to be respected as an adult. Thank you."

Dementia-friendly environments

There are many ways that the environment can be adapted to be less confusing, safer and more comfortable for someone with dementia. A few are listed below. Some of these are based on research carried out at the University of Stirling's Dementia Services Development Centre. See website section, p. 47 for details.

- LIGHTING is very important. As we get older our eyes need more light to see efficiently. Poor lighting can make the person with dementia more confused, and makes falls more likely. Increase light levels, except when and where you want the person to be relaxed or sleep. Exposure to daylight is important too – to boost mood and to help keep the "body clock" working well, which aids night-time sleeping. Pull curtains back and let in as much daylight as possible.

- LIGHT SENSORS can be set up to come on when someone gets out of bed at night. They can be set to switch the bathroom light on, attracting the person towards the toilet. (If possible, arrange the room so that the toilet is visible from the bed.)

- ° Light can cause glare and shadows, which can be confusing for a person with dementia. Avoid shiny floors which can be "misread" as being wet, or shiny tablecloths which can cause glare.

- USE CONTRASTING COLOURS where you want to make things more obvious visually:

  - ° Reduce toileting "accidents" by fitting a contrasting toilet seat to draw attention to the toilet, and help the person see where the edges are.

  - ° Use contrasting colours between the wall and floor to make it obvious where the floor begins.

  - ° Paint handrails and stair rails in contrasting colours to the wall so that they can be easily seen.

  - ° Use contrasting colours for crockery and cutlery, so that each object is clearly defined, and therefore easier to find and use.

- WHEN TO AVOID CONTRASTING COLOURS:

  - ° If wandering is a problem, you can camouflage doors which you don't want the person to use. By painting the wall, the architrave and door the same colour, the door becomes less noticeable.

  - ° Avoid bold patterned shapes or contrasting colours on the carpet, wallpaper or curtains: these can be "misread" and can confuse the person with dementia.

- USE TRADITIONAL FITTINGS – use traditional taps, clearly labelled hot and cold. Some modern designs might not be recognised as being taps.

- BE AWARE OF MIRRORS – in the late stages of dementia, a person may not recognise him/herself in the mirror and may think there is a stranger in the room. If this is a problem, make sure mirrors are covered or removed.

- HELPFUL TECHNOLOGY – it is worth considering some of the numerous products which can make life easier and safer:

  - You could ask your pharmacist about having medicines delivered in pre-packed doses, marked for days of the week and times of day. Automatic pill dispensers, with beep alarms, are also available.

  - There are special plugs which prevent the water overflowing if a tap is left on and which change colour to alert the user that the water is too hot.

  - Electric and gas cookers can be fitted with cut-out mechanisms.

  - "Item locators" can help find a lost wallet or glasses.

  - If wandering is a problem, make sure the person with dementia always carries ID with emergency numbers. Various "tracking" devices are available that can locate someone if they have got lost.

Dementia – facts and figures

Dementia is not a single illness: the term describes a group of symptoms caused by various diseases which damage the brain.

- According to the Alzheimer's Society, in 2012 there were 800,000 people in the UK living with dementia. That number will increase to least a million people by 2021. In the USA, according to the Alzheimer's Association, in 2012 there were 5.4 million people with dementia.

- The symptoms of dementia include memory loss, mood changes and problems with understanding, reasoning and communication. The particular symptoms experienced depend on which condition is causing dementia.

- Although dementia is not a normal part of ageing, it mainly affects older people. One in six people over the age of 80 have dementia. A small percentage of younger people can get it too.

- Two out of three people with dementia are women.

- Most forms of dementia are not inherited, and if your parents develop dementia in old age, there is only a slight increase in risk of you developing it.

- Dementia can affect anybody – men and women, people who have spent their life working with their hands or people who worked more with their brains. Even people such as Iris Murdoch and Terry Pratchett, best-selling authors with brilliant, creative minds, can be affected by it.

- There is as yet no cure, but research is continuing into drugs, vaccines and other possible treatments.

- Research suggests that eating healthily, exercising regularly, drinking only in moderation, not smoking, and keeping socially and mentally active into old age may reduce the risk of developing Alzheimer's disease and vascular dementia.

Different types of dementia

ALZHEIMER'S DISEASE (AD)

The most common cause of dementia is Alzheimer's disease, named after the German neurologist Alois Alzheimer. More than half of all people suffering from dementia have Alzheimer's disease. Chemical and structural changes occur in the brain, so the brain becomes increasingly damaged. A protein called amyloid builds up deposits known as "plaques". "Tangles" of filaments develop, killing brain cells. Although there is no cure, some medicines can temporarily slow down the progression of Alzheimer's disease in some people.

VASCULAR DEMENTIA

After Alzheimer's disease, the second most common form of dementia is vascular dementia (an umbrella term for various types of dementia caused by problems with the vascular system). The vascular system is the blood supply system: if the blood supply to the brain is disrupted – because of a stroke, a series of mini-strokes or damage to the tiny blood vessels deep in the brain – brain cells die, which can lead to vascular dementia. Conditions such as high blood pressure, heart problems, high cholesterol and diabetes can increase the likelihood of this type of dementia, and need to be treated. The progression of vascular dementia differs from that of Alzheimer's: instead of a gradual decline, deterioration happens in steps – symptoms usually remain constant for a while, then suddenly become more severe.

MIXED DEMENTIA

Some people may have more than one type of dementia, for example, Alzheimer's disease and vascular dementia. This is called mixed dementia.

POSTERIOR CORTICAL ATROPHY (PCA)

This is a type of Alzheimer's disease which affects the back of the brain, where visual processing takes place. People suffering from PCA lose the ability to recognise colours, shapes and faces, and the written word. Memory loss often develops only once the disease has progressed. This is the type of Alzheimer's that the author Terry Pratchett has.

DEMENTIA WITH LEWY BODIES (DLB)

About 10 per cent of older people with dementia have dementia with Lewy bodies. Lewy bodies (named after the doctor who discovered them) are tiny deposits of protein that develop in the nerve cells, damaging the brain. Lewy bodies are also found in the brains of people with Parkinson's disease: people with DLB often have symptoms of both Alzheimer's (such as loss of memory and reasoning skills) and Parkinson's (such as stiffness and tremor). They also often experience visual hallucinations – seeing things that are not there in reality.

FRONTO-TEMPORAL DEMENTIA

Fronto-temporal dementia is a relatively rare form of dementia. It can be caused by a range of conditions that damage the frontal and/or temporal lobe (the front and/or the sides of the brain). These are the areas concerned with behaviour, emotion and language, and symptoms of fronto-temporal dementia include changes in behaviour (such as starting to behave in an inappropriate, uninhibited way) and language difficulties. Fronto-temporal dementias are associated with people under the age of 65, and in about a third to a half of cases, the condition runs in families. In its later stages, the symptoms are similar to Alzheimer's disease.

DOWN'S SYNDROME

People with Down's Syndrome are at risk of developing dementia. About 50 per cent of people with Down's Syndrome in their 60s have Alzheimer's disease.

Getting help

Recommended organisations and websites

If you are caring for someone with dementia, you need help. You do not need to try to cope alone. As well as getting help from family and friends, you can access information and support from many sources including health services, social services and voluntary organisations. You can use the websites below to get information and advice, and to find out about carers' support groups in your area.

UK

Alzheimer's Society
Devon House
58 St Katharine's Way
London
E1W 1LB
Helpline: 0300 222 1122
Main switchboard: 020 7423 3500
Email: enquiries@alzheimers.org.uk
Website: www.alzheimers.org.uk

Alzheimer's Society (Wales)
16 Columbus Walk
Atlantic Wharf
Cardiff
CF10 4BY
Phone: 02920 480593

Alzheimer's Society (Northern Ireland)
Unit 4 Balmoral Business Park
Boucher Crescent
Belfast
BT12 6HU
Helpline: 028 90664100
Email: nir@alzheimers.org.uk

Alzheimer Scotland
22 Drumsheugh Gardens
Edinburgh
EH3 7RN
Helpline: 0808 808 3000
Phone: 0131 243 1453
Email: alzheimer@alzscot.org
Website: www.alzscot.org

Dementia Services Development Centre
Iris Murdoch Building
University of Stirling
Stirling
FK9 4LA
Phone: 01786 467740
Website: www.dementia.stir.ac.uk
(On this website you can take a very useful virtual tour of dementia-friendly room designs.)

Republic of Ireland
The Alzheimer Society of Ireland
National Office
Temple Road
Blackrock
Co Dublin
Helpline: 1 800 341 341
Phone: (01) 207 3800
Email: helpline@alzheimer.ie
Website: www.alzheimer.ie

USA
Alzheimer's Association
Alzheimer's Association National Office
225 N. Michigan Ave., Fl. 17
Chicago
IL 60601
Journal: *Alzheimer's & Dementia: The Journal of the Alzheimer's Association*
24/7 Helpline: 1.800.272.3900
Website: www.alz.org

Canada

Alzheimer Society of Canada

20 Eglinton Avenue West, 16th Floor
Toronto
Ontario
M4R 1K8
(There are offices in every province across Canada: see main website
for details.)
Phone: 416-488-8772
Toll-free (from Canada): 1-800-616-8816
Email: info@alzheimer.ca
Website: www.alzheimer.ca

Australia

Alzheimer's Australia

Australia National Office
1 Frewin Place
Scullin
ACT, 2614
National Dementia Helpline: 1800 100 500
Phone: (02) 6254 4233
Email: nat.admin@alzheimers.org.au
Website: www.fightdementia.org.au

New Zealand

Alzheimers New Zealand

National Office
4–12 Cruickshank St
PO Box 14768
Kilbirnie
Wellington 6241
For dementia support: 0800 004 001
Phone: 04 387 8264
Email: nationaloffice@alzheimers.org.nz
Website: www.alzheimers.org.nz